GET OUT OF THE
DIET TRAP

GET OUT OF THE DIET TRAP

Enjoy Eating Again Without Remorse—
A Commonsense Guide to Natural
Weight Control

Walter A. Hans

To order additional copies of this book, contact:
Xlibris Corporation
1-888-795-4274
www.Xlibris.com
Orders@Xlibris.com
40515

CONTENTS

FOREWORD

I've known Walter my entire life. He's my father.

He's not a doctor, a nutritionist, a therapist or a self-proclaimed diet guru. He is an engineer by trade. And, like just about everyone I know, he is concerned about his health and the health of those he loves.

As an engineer, a man of science, and a naturally curious individual, he has always tried to educate himself in the way all things work, so that he could go through life making the most informed decisions possible while obtaining the best desired outcome. A trait, I am happy to report, he has instilled in me as well.

So it was surprising to me that after living a very honest and active life, my Dad still found himself struggling with a weight problem, and eventually discovered he needed coronary bypass surgery!

Knowing my father as I did, and knowing that health was always of great importance to him, this didn't add up. Why wasn't my father at optimum health for his age? This was not a man of indulgences or weak will. He had always taken care of himself. How could this have happened?

It turns out my father was as perplexed as myself and the rest of the family. He had done research and followed the advice of health professionals for as long as I could remember. What had gone wrong?

My father, true to his nature, decided to analyze the problem. But into his research into health and nutrition, he discovered volumes upon volumes of conflicting data. Hundreds of medical and nutritional experts, unable to even distinguish the difference between a healthy lifestyle—and a deadly one!

My father was stymied. How could an entire field of experts not be able to come to even the simplest of concurring conclusions? There had to be an explanation to all of this. Surely the process of keeping the body healthy and alive had to be relatively simple, didn't it? Otherwise, the human race would have been extinct eons ago.

Upon this realization, my father set off on finding a simple, scientific solution for obtaining and maintaining a healthy human body.

No gimmicks, diet tricks or meal plans. No special recipes or taboo foods. Just a simple life philosophy that has been employed by humans since before the term "calorie" was even invented.

The result of these rediscovered epiphanies are bound together in this simple, straightforward book.

Enjoy.

Michael Arthur Hans

CHAPTER 1

YOU ARE WHAT YOU DON'T EAT

"You are what you eat" is a well-known phrase. "You are what you *don't* eat" is a play with words. But what is it supposed to mean? Let me demonstrate it by telling you the following story:

A man (we'll call him Bill) is in his early thirties. He works out regularly; his weight is ideal, he feels healthy, he is successful, and he enjoys life. He mostly eats on the run because he lives a busy life.

One day Bill gets a minor infection. His body's immune system needs specific nutrients to fight the infection. The body cannot find the nutrients it needs in the food Bill eats. The body searches for organs it can deplete. First, it depletes less critical and then more critical organs.

The infection is cured, and the body now wants to replace the nutrients it took from the organs it had depleted. In search for the needed nutrients, the body causes Bill to keep on eating after he is satisfied. He has cravings.

Bill keeps on eating the same food he ate before, just more of it. He overeats. Bill slowly gains weight, and working out becomes more and more of a chore. He takes pills that promise to boost his strength, and he overextends himself. He stops working out, keeps on overeating, and, as a result, gains more weight.

Bill takes appetite suppressors and gets indigestion. Certain foods don't seem to agree with him anymore. He stops eating them.

Overweight is now affecting his lifestyle. He goes on a diet. Bill is being told what foods he is "allowed" to eat because some foods are "bad" for him. Most of the foods he used to eat are not good for him anymore. Bill now eats a lot of food substitutes.

Bill's body still has not found the nutrients it needs to stay healthy. His cholesterol levels are high. The doctor puts Bill on a low-fat diet. He now eats margarine (which Bill dislikes) instead of butter.

Bill's cravings have become worse. He secretly eats cake and ice cream. He tries to count calories without much success. Nevertheless, Bill knows that he cannot afford to eat fruits or vegetables after an ice cream binge or he will exceed his daily calorie "allowance." He is also not excited at all about having to eat string beans after he had eaten ice cream.

Bill has just been told that he needs major heart surgery because his arteries are clogged.

Then Bill wakes up. It was all a bad dream!

Or was it? Have you had a similar experience?

Do you really want to be told what you are "allowed" to eat, or use drugs and procedures that inhibit proper digestion, risking well-being and longevity just to lose weight?

Do you wish you could

- ➢ feel and look good, have the energy to do what you like?
- ➢ stay healthy and young?
- ➢ enjoy eating and eat the foods you like?

If you eat the foods you really like, in moderation, all this is likely to happen. Your body needs a wide range of nutrients to function. It only gets these nutrients from the food you eat or drink.

At the time of this writing there were over twenty-eight thousand diet books listed on Amazon.com. If you were able to read them all, you would probably be totally confused and scared out of eating altogether. Magazines are full of advice: what to eat and what not to eat. Television bombards you with nutritional advice day and night. Anybody can offer advice and often does.

Misinformation has gone rampant. Be critical! Be very critical! Your life may depend upon it!

Is it surprising that more and more people don't eat right? Do you? I did not and I gained weight. Experimenting with so-called weight loss diets eventually caused my weight to go out of control. I have since been able to lose excess weight and keep it off. I have been using common sense. Eating has become pure joy again.

I wrote this book to share my success with you. If my conclusions make sense to you, great! If reading this book inspires you to find your own way to success that would be even better.

Chapter 2

The Problem

You may not remember it, but as a baby, you knew when to eat and when to stop eating. You made yourself heard when it was time to eat and nobody could get more food into your mouth when your hunger was satisfied. You did not miss the nutrients you needed; they were all in mother's milk—nature's formula.

Maybe your trouble started as a child when nature's formula was replaced with formulas that came in a bottle, a can, or a jar.

Let's assume that scientists are able to analyze all the nutrients, which are included in the mother's milk. Let's further assume that these nutrients can be readily duplicated in a manufactured formula and that the formula includes all of them.

Manufactured foods have to be preserved. The preservation process is a compromise between preventing spoilage (e.g., pasteurization) and not destroying the nutrients in the process. Nutrients do not always win in the compromise.

Maybe your troubles started as a child when you were rewarded with a candy.

Eating food with added sugar (not naturally found in foods such as fruits) makes the food that is good for you, such as fruits and vegetables, taste bland and undesirable. The sweetness of refined sugar or syrup is so strong; it impedes your appetite. Who wants to eat spinach after eating ice cream, cake, pudding, or drinking soda?

Maybe your troubles started when you went on your first weight loss diet.

Why Don't Weight Loss Diets Work for You?

A limited choice in the food available to you or the complex task of selecting and preparing food may limit the variety of food you are normally eating. You may not get all the nutrients your body needs. This alone can cause weight gain because the body urges you to keep on eating until it finds the nutrients it needs. You have cravings.

More likely, a change in your eating habits in your nutritional requirements or in the quality and consistency of the food you are eating causes an imbalance between your body's needs for specific nutrients and the supply of those nutrients. There are many circumstances that can trigger such imbalances.

It really gets dangerous when you start eliminating some so-called bad foods, just because a weight loss diet says so.

The exclusion or partial avoidance of individual foods or whole food groups limits the nutrients available to your body. The lack of important nutrients causes you to be undernourished no matter how much you eat.

Diet remedies, recommended for weight loss, may not always specifically tell you to limit the range of nutrients in your diet. Nevertheless, the regimen these remedies require may make you consciously or subconsciously avoid certain types of food or whole food groups.

If you had cravings before you went on a diet that limits food choices, these cravings will become worse once you are on the diet. You are in a trap—the Diet Trap.

Suffering and not losing weight, or regaining it, may be the least of your problems. You may be ruining your health.

Your body has simple and unmistakable indicators that tell you when, how much, and what to eat. If you let your instincts guide you, the body will do the rest.

There is no logical reason why you can't do again what once was so easy to do, unless you are caught in a trap. And this is exactly what happens when you start substituting instinct or common sense with unnatural regimens (diet fads).

According to newspaper and magazine articles, overweight is entirely your fault. You eat too much, you eat food that is "bad" for you, and you don't get enough exercise. Benevolently, some articles let you blame the fast-food restaurants, your school, or your parents. This wisdom will not help you nor solve the obesity crisis—and neither will social pressure.

Social Pressure

We are creatures of habit, formed by upbringing, social rules, and other outside influences. We do what our mother says, the doctor says, books and magazines say, and what advertisers say. We do what others say, often without being aware or critical of it.

Eating has become a compulsion for some of us. We eat,

- ➢ when it is "time" to eat;
- ➢ when we are told to eat;
- ➢ when we celebrate;
- ➢ when we feel good;
- ➢ when we feel bad, lonely, or sad;
- ➢ when we are nervous;
- ➢ when we want to get tired;
- ➢ when we are tired;
- ➢ when we work, go to the movies, go to a ball game, watch television; and
- ➢ when we are anywhere, with anybody, anytime.

We are busy. We are eating fast because we don't have time to eat. Eating on the run causes indigestion. Our belly hurts. When it stops hurting, it must be time to eat again. Indigestion becomes a way of life.

The Vicious Cycle

As we all know, a simple solution to lose excess weight would be to stop overeating. What keeps us from doing that? The following is a typical sequence:

1. A change in our eating habits or other influences deprives us of specific nutrients, which the body needs.
2. Cravings tell us to keep on eating in search for those nutrients.
3. We gain weight as a result of overeating.
4. Social pressure and medical advice compel us to lose weight.
5. We go on a diet, and we change our eating habits *again* without being aware of the changes that made us gain weight in the first place.

In search for a way to lose weight, we find weight loss diets that make us (intentionally or unintentionally) limit the variety of food we are eating without properly addressing the need for the nutrients we are missing. As a result, we experience even stronger cravings than those that made us overeat in the first place.

Being overweight slows us down. We start to burn less energy. Eventually, eating seems to be the only thing left that is fun to do. Now we are trapped, and we are feeling guilty because everybody tells us that the only pleasure left to us is bad for us.

Where Did We Go Wrong?

It takes years to gain a substantial amount of weight. With all those promises out there for a quick loss of many pounds, we don't see any reason for alarm when we notice that our body starts storing fat. We believe that we can lose weight anytime we want to. Gaining weight can actually become appealing; we join a growing majority. We can boast that we are going on a diet like everybody else.

It is comforting to have friends who encourage us and who are willing to join us in being "bad." We get all excited when we get together and eat food that is "sooo good." This food is usually loaded with sugar and fat.

There will probably be no ill effect if we overeat once in a while, but when it becomes a habit or compulsion, we gain weight.

The tragedy starts when we decide that the time has come to lose weight seriously. Then we realize that all those promises of easy weight loss don't seem to work for us. They may work initially, but the regimen becomes unbearable after a while and the weight starts coming back.

Failure to lose weight turns into guilt, and guilt turns into depression. Now we have to overeat to save our sanity.

Eating has to be a pleasure and not drudgery. Counting calories, grams of carbohydrates, percentages of fat, and eating food we don't like is an annoyance at best.

The worst part about most weight loss diets is the fact that they lead us away from our instincts, from our natural ability to eat what the body needs. Natural indicators are being replaced with unnatural regimens.

Nutritional experts attack each other's theories with passion. Only one can be right in any specific matter. Assuming he is right, logic tells us that everyone else, all of these so-called experts are wrong!

CHAPTER 3

A SENSIBLE SOLUTION

Theory:

What Should You Do?

If you are comfortable with your weight and your looks, chances are you don't have a weight problem.

The picture you see in the magazine of another person may look good, but that person is not you. You may look better and a lot sexier than what you think. When you get older, a healthy overweight will hide some wrinkles and may fit your lifestyle.

If you are uncomfortable with your weight, you don't have to be miserable and sacrifice the fun of eating. You just have to heighten your awareness to the level you once had, before your eating habits changed. You most likely had this awareness level as a child before you were forced to finish your plate or were given candies, cookies, and soda as a treat or a reward. You had this awareness level before you were told what to eat and what not to eat.

Only you can help yourself. Eating is a personal matter. Use common sense and follow your instincts. Interfering with your instincts is asking for trouble.

Your body tells you when you are doing things right. It makes you feel good. Your body will even tell you when you are going in the right direction. When you eat the right food and don't overeat, you feel better immediately. You are less tired, have less abdominal pains, and feel a spurt of energy.

After many years of government guidelines and medical or not-so-medical advice on how to eat right, obesity in the United States has reached epidemic proportions. Estimates vary widely. According to government reports, nearly 60 percent of adults are overweight or obese, as are nearly 13 percent of children.

Considering the impact of obesity on productivity, health care costs (estimated to be $93 billion per year) and the quality of life, these developments are nothing short of a national crisis.

How to Follow Your Instincts?

The human body needs a steady flow of nutrients, motion, and rest to function and to stay healthy. Instincts regulate this flow through the pleasure/pain stimulus. The body's needs depend upon its size, condition, and exposure. These needs change all the time.

Matching the body's needs gives us the greatest sensation of comfort, happiness, and pleasure. Any mismatch, too much or too little, causes discomfort and pain.

The excessive pursuit of pleasure, in all of its forms, usually causes disillusionment or pain. The consequences of drug abuse—legal or not—are a perfect example. Abstinence also causes suffering, if natural instincts are being suppressed.

Our ability to learn, remember, and reason increases our chances for survival. It can also lead us away from following our instincts. A baby will let us know when it is feeding time. But the baby will spit out the food we are forcing into his or her mouth when the hunger is satisfied.

Science has found many reasons why people gain excess weight as they grow older. The fact that a large number of people never gain excess weight seems to make these reasons look more like excuses. People, whose weight is considered normal, do not need instructions when to eat, how much to eat, what to eat, or what not to eat. They control their weight without effort by following their instincts.

What are these instincts, and how can we follow them? Hunger and appetite are signals we are getting from our body. These are the instincts that regulate our food intake.

What is hunger?

Hunger is a feeling of emptiness and even pain, the need of restoring energy. Hunger tells us when to eat.

What is appetite?

Appetite is the appeal of certain foods, a preference of some foods over others. Appetite tells us what to eat.

Hunger is the stronger of the two instincts. It cannot be suppressed. Appetite can be suppressed. The suppression of appetite deprives us of the ability to choose the nutrients the body needs. Environmental influences, sickness, physical and emotional stress can cause nutritional imbalances. The inability to respond to changing nutritional requirements can cause the body to become undernourished no matter how much we are eating. An insufficient supply of the nutrients, needed by the body at any given time, causes cravings.

What are cravings?

Cravings are the strong desire to eat or keep on eating, a longing for more food when we are actually satisfied (full). Cravings tell us that the body is not getting the nutrients it needs.

Cravings are an indication that the food we are eating does not include all the nutritional elements the body needs. Cravings interfere with and obstruct the hunger instinct. It is the body's way to search for the missing nutrients. Cravings make us overeat, and overeating is the most common cause of being overweight.

My Hypothesis

Proper eating habits are essential for good health and survival. Eating and drinking support all functions of the body by supplying the necessary nutrients.

I have posted the following hypothesis for the experts, either for them to investigate further or simply to mock.

Our body guides us in the selection of food and the quantity we should be eating without requiring a conscious effort, if we follow the instinctive indicators of hunger and appetite.

Any interference with the body's ability to regulate the food intake, such as food shortages, environmental influences, sickness, and physical or emotional stress can cause nutritional imbalances. Drugs, as well as dietary regimens, which interfere with the body's instincts, can prolong nutritional imbalances and even be the cause of them through suppression of the appetite and hunger indicators.

Our body, in its search for missing nutrients, may cause us to overeat through a stimulus called cravings. Prolonged overeating leads to overweight and obesity.

This trend can be reversed, and a proper weight balance can be restored through heightened awareness of the body's instinctive indicators. Hunger and appetite regulate the amount of food we are eating and our selection of food through the pain/pleasure stimulus. We experience pain if we do not select the proper types of food or eat the wrong amounts. Following our instincts makes eating a pleasure and promotes a feeling of well-being.

Early in our life almost all of us have been able to maintain a perfect weight balance without any conscious effort—most babies know instinctively how much to eat. If our body was able to balance its weight before it started to gain excess weight, it is logical that our body can do it again.

Selecting small portions from a wide range of nutritious, unadulterated food, whenever we are hungry, is the best insurance for getting the proper nutrients needed to support our health without gaining excess weight.

Eating a large variety of food in small portions increases the probability that we are supplying the body with a large variety of nutrients, those that are known as well as those that are still unknown. The more nutrients available to the body, the more likely it is that the body will stay strong, healthy, painless, and young.

Practice:

My Experience

As a child, I was diagnosed as being undernourished. I was a victim of starvation. Trust me—overweight is the lesser of the two evils. Once food became plentiful again, my weight fortunately normalized.

I love to eat, and I love to eat well. Rich foods are my favorites. I learned how to cook to assure that I can eat what I like, whenever I want to. All my life I have worked hard, and stress is no stranger to me. Stress makes me want to eat.

I moved a lot in my twenties and early thirties. I moved from country to country and from city to city. Changes in the types of food available had an obvious effect on my weight. I noticed a slight weight gain almost every time I moved.

Eventually, I became weight conscious, and it was time to lose weight. Eliminating foods sweetened with refined sugar or syrup did the trick for a while. I would lose a few pounds and get back into my comfort range.

When I got older, the excess weight shifted to my belly. Any weight gain now became uncomfortable, and losing weight became more difficult. I turned to a "low-carbohydrate diet," and that seemed to be the answer—for a while.

Although I love protein-type foods, life became monotonous. Even the foods you like become boring if you eat them a lot and especially if you are limited to them. Eating mainly proteins (and probably not enough of a variety of foods) caused strong cravings.

Carbohydrates suddenly became my favorite foods. I got those cravings for pasta, bread, and all the other foods rich in carbohydrates. I felt bad that I could not eat them in sufficient quantities, and I felt worse when I did. I found myself eating fats in large quantities to stop the cravings.

I had subconsciously come to the conclusion that about everything I ate was bad for me, and I felt bad every time I would eat. I had the combined knowledge of all those diet recommendations and exclusions that are bombarding us daily, and I was totally confused. I was also gaining weight, and there seemed to be no way to stop it. Indigestion had become a way of life.

When my weight had risen to about thirty-five pounds above my comfort range, I had to find a way to lose weight without regaining it. The only other option was slowing down to avoid exertion. Slowing down was not an option for me. Unnatural eating regimens and living a miserable life was not acceptable. Eating had once been a pleasure for me, and I was determined to make it a pleasure again.

Not a single diet had worked for me. Losing weight was not the problem. Keeping it off was.

I recognized that the harder I tried to lose weight, the harder it seemed to get. I tried to remember what I did to control my weight before I had weight problems. I remembered that I did not have to control my weight. Eating was a natural thing. I suddenly realized that my problems started when I read about all those foods I was not supposed to eat.

The obvious answer was to limit the amount of food I was eating. I started by fasting, which lasted less than a day. I then made an effort to eat just as much as necessary to avoid hunger. In order to make eating enjoyable again, I chose a small plate. I put a variety of small pieces of food on the plate and decorated it with all kinds of colorful condiments and tidbits. I chose a small plate in order to create the impression of a "full plate."

I looked at my creation for a while and enjoyed the aroma of the food. Enjoying the aroma and appearance of food is a pleasure, which can definitely be enjoyed without guilt and consequences. I started to eat slowly. I found flavor sensations I had not experienced in a while by chewing the food longer than I usually had done.

After a few bites, the flavor sensation diminished, and I did not feel the urge to eat any longer. I stopped eating. I was satisfied. Eating once again had been fun. After a few hours, I became hungry again, and I repeated the routine.

I lost five pounds during the first week. I had a lot more energy (the feeling of being full was gone), and I was not hungry once. To my surprise, I lost another five pounds in the second week.

Now I got concerned. I was not quite sure what I was doing, and I was worried about losing weight too fast. My initial goal was to lose fifteen pounds. The remaining five pounds I dropped over the next three weeks. I slowed down the weight loss process by eating a bit more than what I needed to satisfy my hunger.

Over the next several months, my work kept me from paying attention to my eating habits, and stress made me eat more than what was needed to satisfy the hunger. I also ate food that was sweetened.

Nevertheless, I maintained the reduced weight level and did not peak by more than three pounds over several months. I did that without any conscious effort. The body took care of itself. Whenever I ate too much, I got this "heavy feeling," and I stopped. Overeating wasn't fun anymore. I had learned to eat in moderation.

I ate a greater variety of food, and eating was fun again. The cravings had stopped. Whenever the cravings came back, I was reminded to return to my routine.

I still had a bulge around my belly, and exercise would just not get rid of it no matter how much I exercised my abdominal muscles. I must have had strong abdominal muscles, but nobody ever knew; the muscles were covered with fat.

A belly is not considered fashionable in our society. It also gets in the way when you bend over, as it slows you down. I had to get rid of it.

I followed my routine now more consciously, and again I managed to lose weight as much as three pounds a week. I can lose one pound a week without even trying. I follow my routine in principle without thinking about it. I eat sweetened foods once in a while. I never stay hungry. Most of all, I enjoy eating and have no reason to feel guilty anymore. Sometimes I eat in a hurry and gulp my food down. Indigestion quickly reminds me to slow down.

The question arose, Was my weight loss actually the result of sensible eating habits, or did other circumstances cause it? Forced overeating answered this question. I immediately gained weight again. But now, I know how to lose weight, and I can keep it low for the rest of my life without gimmicks and without suffering.

How Should You Do It?

This chapter will tell you how to follow your instincts and overcome cravings.

For those looking for a way out of the Diet Trap, as I call it, I am sharing my experiences and thoughts in this book, and I will tell you what has helped me to enjoy eating again without guilt and suffering.

Eating should be a pleasure. Weight control has to be a way of life. Our body tells us how much food and what type of food it needs. The challenge is, How do we know what our body is saying?

Heighten Your Awareness

You were able to control your weight effortlessly at onetime. You followed a simple routine: You ate when you were hungry, and you ate the food you liked. You did that without ever thinking about your weight or what you were doing. How can you get back to this healthy state of mind?

Here are some simple routines that heighten your awareness. They are working for me, and I hope they will work for you.

➤ Chew Well

Chewing is the key to a sensible weight control. Chew well. Chewing is not only one of the most important phases of the digestive process; it helps you to taste the food. It will also help you to avoid indigestion. When you chew a bite about twenty times or more (soft food will take less—the purpose of chewing is to break down the food), you will experience flavors you never knew existed. Go for the flavor!

Please don't count while you are chewing. Don't turn eating into an exercise. Just enjoy it.

You want to get back into healthy eating habits that are effortless? Proper chewing will help you to enjoy every bite. This becomes important when you don't eat much.

If you chew well, you will experience that after about five to ten bites (they can be big ones) you are satisfied. You will have to pay attention. Your cravings may tell you to keep on eating. Everything and everybody you know may tell you to keep on eating.

Just stop after five to ten bites. Get up from the table or just stop eating if it is not socially acceptable to get up. Rest or engage in some activities that will take your mind off the food. Physical activities are good. You will have more energy, and you can use it. If you are still hungry (really hungry after about thirty minutes), have a few more bites. Then stop again.

> ## Take Time to Eat

Take time out for eating. Put your mind on the food whenever you eat. How can you enjoy your food if you don't pay any attention? Take a break and relax. Don't read the paper, watch television, or anything else. Try not to talk while eating.

Don't eat on the run. Even if you grab a quick bite on the street, a hot dog for example, find a quiet corner and focus on your food. Let the traffic go by. You will be much less nervous or tense when you become part of the traffic again.

Business luncheons are bad news. Avoid them if you can. If you cannot avoid them, let other people do most of the talking while you eat very little.

> ## Make Eating a Pleasure

Let every meal (this means whenever you open your mouth to eat) be an occasion. Choose a pleasant surrounding. Set the table, decorate the plate, and garnish it. Enjoy your food first with your eyes before you eat it. Candles, soft music, a well-decorated table, attractive clothing, and pleasant company are not only romantic; these things will make you feel good. Feeling good when you are eating is *vital*.

Small quantities of colorful tidbits, including fruits and vegetables, in a large variety, and well decorated invite you to sample and enjoy. This way of eating is certainly more pleasurable and healthier than sitting in front of the television and eating without being conscious about what you are doing.

The smell and appearance of well-prepared and nicely arranged food is almost as enjoyable as eating it. Good restaurants know that. The decorative presentation of the food is one of the reasons why you want to go back and pay the high prices.

You may not always have the time or the opportunity to celebrate eating.

It is better not to eat than eating in a hurry or without paying attention.

➤ **Make Sure You Eat a Large Variety of Food**

Your appetite will guide you to the nutrients your body needs. Follow your appetite. Include all kinds of food in your menus. Garnish your plate with condiments you like to eat. Serve a variety of foods; include fresh vegetables and fruits. Don't overcook vegetables. Frozen, canned, or dried fruits and vegetables are better than none at all. Eat the foods you like and get to know a few new ones.

Many of us are in a rut. We do not like to experiment or do not have time to bother and, therefore, are eating the same food all the time. This food may not give the body all the nutrients it needs.

You are missing out on a whole segment of the world, that is out there, if you don't experiment and sample new foods. Be curious and not suspicious. It does not hurt to taste new foods. If you don't like them, you do not have to eat them.

Variety Is the Secret to Success

➤ **Think Small**

If you make eating a pleasure and you eat slowly, your body will have a chance to tell you when it is satisfied. You will be able to stop eating after a few bites and feel energetic instead of feeling heavy.

Eating slowly and chewing well will help you to think quality instead of quantity. If you have gotten used to large portions, change that habit. Use a small plate the size of a saucer. Garnish with lettuce, tomato wedges, pickles, a couple of olives, herbs, etc., and you will have a full plate. Feel free to eat the garnish.

You will get the impression that you ate a lot. Who cares if you are kidding yourself? You are kidding yourself if you think that you have to eat a lot!

➤ Enjoy Being Hungry

The feeling of hunger is a sensation that heightens your appreciation for food. Hunger only gets nasty when you ignore it for too long. If you eat when you are hungry, eating will be more of a pleasure.

Your appetite will lead you to the food that is good for you. Do not listen to people who tells you that you cannot eat the food you desire whenever you want to. Do not suppress your appetite.

Any type of food eaten in excess can be harmful. If you eat a large variety of foods and not much of each, you don't have to worry about eating fat or any other of those so-called bad foods. How bad can any regular food be for you if eaten in moderation?

Severe hunger makes us gulp our food. It is best not to wait too long when hunger calls. Eating slowly when hungry can be particularly enjoyable because our senses are on the food.

➤ Don't Mistake Cravings for Hunger

If you feel satisfied after you ate but you still have the urge to keep on eating, you have cravings (see definition at the beginning of this chapter). Cravings are the major reason for overeating. Cravings will diminish once you start increasing the variety of the food you are eating.

In the meantime, you may want to find foods that soothe the cravings. Commercial snacks are often heavily seasoned to make you eat more. You will be able to identify them because you can't stop eating them. Some snack food advertisements even tell you that you won't be able to stop eating them.

Make your own snacks. A piece of sharp cheddar, nonsweetened crackers (if you can find them) and bread sticks, half a boiled egg, fatty foods, and foods with strong flavors do it for me.

Sometimes a glass of water will do the trick. Many people do not drink enough water. Dehydration can cause the urge to eat something moist.

> ## Be Patient

You gained your weight over how many years? As long as you are going in the right direction, you are all right. False ambitions can ruin it for you. Eating may then become what you are trying to avoid—a weight loss diet regimen.

You Have Done It Before; You Can Do It Again

A change of habits does not happen overnight. You will have to pay attention to what you are doing until you are able to do it without thinking. Once you consciously break a few social or dietary eating rules, you will feel better and you are not likely to be ever a slave to these rules again.

Instead of gulping your food, you will instinctively take smaller bites and chew well. It may take a while to establish a routine, but getting there is going in the right direction. If you give your digestive system a rest once in a while, the feeling you get will make you aware that overeating actually causes pain.

The following suggestions may make changing your eating habits easier for you and help you to enjoy eating again.

> ## Do Not Overeat

Once you start improving your eating habits, you will experience a feeling of well-being. You will have more energy because the weight of your full belly and the heavy feeling in your belly are not slowing you down so much anymore.

Chewing breaks down the food for proper digestion. Saliva predigests your food. You will help your digestive system if you chew well.

Cravings suppress the hunger instinct. When you have cravings, you eat until you are full until pain stops you from eating. Living in pain becomes a way of life. Heavy digestion makes you sleepy. You move less and burn less food energy.

If your digestive system is not overloaded with food, it can do a better job. Your stomach will function better if you eat slowly. You can actually feel the joy of anticipation.

➢ Pig Out Once In A While

When you want to lose weight, occasional heavy eating slows the weight loss. But it is important that you do it once in a while. When you are trying to maintain a steady weight, you can eat heavily once a week without any problem. You will know when it is time to get serious again.

Knowing that you can pig out does not make it so desirable anymore.

After you have changed your eating habits for a while, you will lose the urge to eat heavily. You will now quickly recognize that overeating makes you tired and causes pain. Letting your instincts tell you when and how much to eat becomes an enjoyable habit.

➢ Don't Drink while Eating

Drinks dilute your digestive juices and can spoil your appetite, especially with sugared drinks. Drink before you start eating if you are thirsty. When you select your food well and you chew it well, you should not get thirsty.

Wine is considered to be good for the digestion. It also enables you to eat more. Have the wine after you had a chance to digest the food somewhat. Do not drink alcohol directly before eating. The effect of the alcohol will diminish your ability to taste your food fully, and you will overeat without noticing. You can be more liberal if you are only maintaining your weight.

➤ Watch That Sugar

My experience has been that eating or drinking food with added sugar (not naturally found in foods such as fruits) makes you crave for more sugar. When you come down from your sugar high, you will only be satisfied when you ingest more sugar. It is addictive.

Because the sweetness of refined sugar or syrup is so strong, it impedes the appetite. It makes other foods taste bland. Refined sugar impedes the desire to eat fruits, vegetables, and other foods with high nutritional values. Fruit sugar, which is not addictive, loses its appeal. Cravings will not be far behind.

You can break that spell. After about two days without added sugar in your food, you will feel less of a craving for sweetened food. After a week, the cravings will be gone. Thereafter, the first bite of something sugared tastes disgustingly sweet; take a second bite and you are addicted again.

Avoid foods with added sugar if you want to lose weight. Some sugar is okay if you are maintaining your weight and you can control yourself. Artificial sweeteners are just as bad as sugar—without the fun. Although artificial sweeteners do not contain any food energy, they tease you into eating more. Fruit sugar, a natural part of fruits, is okay; but eat fruits in bites (not whole fruits at a time) if you want to lose weight.

➤ Cover All Your Bases

Make sure that you eat all of the main nutrients, such as carbohydrates, proteins, and fat. Take it easy with carbohydrates, but make sure you include them. Adding carbohydrates and fat to your diet is more satisfying and may make you less hungry. It also makes eating more fun. If you eat small portions, you don't have to count calories.

Daily Scorecard

You don't need this scorecard to succeed. All you have to do is eat a large variety of foods, in small portions, enjoy eating, and watch your weight normalize. Nevertheless, this scorecard may help you to get started. Fill out this scorecard at the end of the day.

Enter the following numbers under SCORE:

> 0—If you did not think about the subject
> 1—If you considered the subject but are not sure how well you did
> 2—If you were successful at least once during the day
> 3—If you were successful more than once during the day

SUBJECT	SCORE
I only ate whenever I started to feel really hungry.	
I used a small dish and arranged the food attractively.	
I ate small portions of a variety of food.	
I ate what my appetite told me and not what I was "supposed" to eat.	
I chewed well and enjoyed every bite.	
I stopped eating when the hunger stopped.	
I ate in a quiet, pleasant place without distractions.	
I did not drink while eating.	
I did not eat anything sweetened.	
I did not give in to cravings.	
Total Score	

If your totalscore is

0	Don't give up! There is always tomorrow.
1-5	You did something right—you got started!
6-10	You are on your way, and you are going in the right direction.
11-15	You don't have to feel guilty anymore.
16-20	You are getting your weight under control
21-25	You have more energy now; use it to do the things you like!
26-30	You know how to lose weight now, anytime you wish.

CHAPTER 4

SOME ADVICE

How Fast Can You Lose Weight?

If you are considerably overweight, it probably took you several years to gain it all. Chances are you have tried weight loss diets without much success. You lost weight several times and gained it all back and then some. It is understandable that you have become impatient, and you may be even desperate. But forcing weight loss may not be healthy, and you are much more likely to fail.

If losing weight is important to you, keeping the weight off once you have lost it is even more important. Sudden weight loss, except for the first few pounds, is not healthy and not sustainable without serious consequences. Vital organs can be damaged if important nutrients are withheld for an extended time.

My own experiences may give you an indication of what can be done. I started to eat very little, and I was able to lose five pounds during the first week. I lost another five pounds in the second week.

My initial goal was to lose fifteen pounds. After the first two weeks I purposely ate a bit more than what I needed to satisfy my hunger. The remaining five pounds I lost over the next three weeks.

Over the next several months, my work kept me from paying attention to my eating habits. Nevertheless, whenever I ate too much, I got this full feeling, and I stopped eating. Overeating was not enjoyable anymore. I also noticed that the cravings had stopped. I maintained the reduced weight level and did not peak by more than three pounds. I did that without any conscious effort. The body took care of itself.

I have since managed to lose more weight slowly in the right places. I have lost as much as three pounds a week (one pound a week without any special effort).

I follow my routine without thinking much about it. I eat sweetened foods once in a while, and I never stay hungry. Most of all, I enjoy eating and have no reason to feel guilty anymore.

Be patient. If you try too hard, you will suffer. Suffering will lead you astray and before you know, you will be back to your old habits and begin to gain weight again.

How to Get Started?

Just order from my catalogue of high-priced food substitutes!

I'm kidding, of course.

It is not a matter of starting something; it is a matter of stopping bad eating practices. Eating a large variety of foods, in small portions, whenever you are hungry is not something that takes a lot of willpower or preparation. You can ease into it.

You choose the food you like and eat it. Just follow your appetite. What is good for me is not necessarily good for you. Trusting your instincts may first be a bit difficult, especially if you have been counting calories for years—but it works.

Your ideal weight is what you think it is. Don't worry about what the experts are saying. Everybody is different.

Use common sense and follow your instincts if you have a strong desire to look good, feel good, enjoy your food, and have a lot of energy.

The suggestions in Chapters 3 and 4 may help you to find your way. You are taking a large step toward weight loss if you eat whatever you feel like eating, chew well, and stop eating after a few bites.

Fasting will kick-start your weight loss. Fasting helps you to distinguish between hunger and cravings. It also puts your mind on the food while you are eating. You do not have to stop eating altogether. Drink a lot of water, have a cracker (without sugar) when it gets real bad. Have some cheese, an olive if you like it, something salty or fatty. Chew the food well.

Keep food out of sight. Keep yourself busy. If you don't think about food, you won't eat any.

How to Live In a Large-Portion World

Have you noticed that it has become very difficult to buy or order food in small portions? Some restaurants are famous for their big portions. All-you-can-eat restaurants are mushrooming across the country. What can you do?

Having fun eating at home makes restaurants less attractive, and you can save money.

You do not have to go to all-you-can-eat restaurants unless you really want to pig out. If you go to a fast-food restaurant, skip the soda and eat a small meal slowly. Do not eat while driving. When you get your food at the drive-through window, stop and eat before you drive on. It is safer and avoids indigestion.

Some fast-food restaurants now have salads or side dishes you can combine for a meal. Order the regular-sized burger and not the "quadruple meat whammy."

Disagree with the Social Eating Rules.

When you are invited to a restaurant, you have a number of choices:

1. You can make it your pig-out day (day of unrestricted eating), and eat whatever and as much as you wish.

2. Many people already eat salads when they go to a restaurant. When you chew your salad well, a small portion will satisfy you. But don't skimp on the dressing, eat a reasonable amount of any dressing you like (forget the boring no-fat dressings). Remember, it is important to enjoy eating.

3. Sometimes there are appetizers on the menu that you can eat as a main meal. They are usually portioned sensibly, like a smaller main course. Say no when the waiter asks you if you wish to have the appetizer in a main course portion.

4. If you don't feel like eating an appetizer, order the main course without the extras, eat some of the meat or fish, nibble on the sides, and take the rest home. At home, you can portion the food and freeze it for future days.

5. When you live in hotels a lot, choose those that offer efficiencies. Having a stove and a refrigerator (and some cooking skills) keeps you out of the restaurants. Convenience stores and supermarkets now have salads, soups, and cooked meals that you can eat in your hotel room. Pizza is not bad for you if you buy it by the piece.

When you prepare your own food, try to buy and cook in small quantities. You can buy and cook in large quantities but store the food in small portions.

Stores will reapportion any store-packaged food for you. All you have to do is ask. Most fresh food, including bread can be portioned and frozen. Canned food may be portioned and will last for a while in the refrigerator.

Dry soups, for example, can be portioned. The leftovers of fresh vegetables or fruits usually last a few days if you clean them and store them in the refrigerator. Summer sausage, cheese, and foods in jars make good snacks, and they last for a while.

Having food preserved in small portions has the advantage that you can now compose an impressive meal with different kinds of foods anytime you want. Always have garnish on hand—it's appetizing and colorful.

The money you waste when you overeat can be used to buy fancy tidbit food such as caviar, pate, exotic mushrooms, anything pickled, and whatever else you can find that you like in a posh food store.

You can prepare fancy food items yourself and preserve them in portions. If you don't know how to cook, go and learn how to cook. Cooking is almost as much fun as eating. Any of your favorite foods will now be at your fingertips anytime you get hungry.

Eating will never be boring again.

Don't Play the Yo-Yo Game

Some people are eating a lot in preparation of going on a weight loss diet, and they are eating a lot after they failed to stay on that diet; I call this the yo-yo game.

How often have you heard, "I want to have fun before I go on a diet"? Maybe you've said it to yourself.

Many weight loss diets require sacrifices, which are,

- ➢ painful (not enough food);
- ➢ boring (bland foods);
- ➢ tedious (special foods); and
- ➢ unhealthy (limited variety of foods).

Sacrifice cannot be sustained for any length of time with all the temptations around us. Sacrifice, therefore, usually ends in failure and disappointment. Weight loss diets do not always solve the problem that made us gain weight in the first place. They often make it worse. The excess weight will come back soon after the diet becomes unbearable. Unsuccessful weight loss diets may be the main reason for the overweight epidemic.

"I was not able to stay on the diet, I am depressed. I have to eat"!

Overeating before we go on a diet and overeating after we abandon the diet because we are depressed usually results in a net weight gain.

Suggestions How to Lose Weight Are Endless

"Buy this exercise machine and you will lose weight!"

Sure you will but only if the energy you get from the food you eat is less than the energy you burn.

Everybody is a weight loss expert as long as they can count. "Only one percent of fat, only two grams of carbohydrates, only thirty calories, and you will lose weight."

Sure you will but only if the energy you get from the food you eat is less than the energy you burn.

Follow the wisdom you can get from magazines, books, television, the Internet, and even cereal boxes and you will lose weight.

Sure you will but only if the energy you get from the food you eat is less than the energy you burn.

Whenever you change your eating habits, you will probably lose some weight. The body has to adjust and get the necessary nutrients from other sources. Your body needs time to adjust. You may also be eating less. Once your body adjusts, the weight loss will stop quickly.

Have you ever wondered why these big weight loss diets can pay millions of dollars for advertising year after year? If these diets would solve weight problems, wouldn't they have sold themselves out of business by now?

At the time this book was written, there were over twenty-eight thousand diet books listed on Amazon.com. Magazines are filled with suggestions on how to lose weight. The Internet is cluttered with drug and diet food solicitations. Television has many shows devoted to weight control.

Weight loss medications are being advertised more and more frequently. These medications claim that they will burn your fat, prevent you from digesting your food, or obscure your appetite. Let's assume they really work—what will that do to your health?

Distractions Can Make It Difficult

Our lifestyle is reflected in the things that surround us. The things we like are usually nearby and easy to reach. We go to places that cater to our wishes, and we meet with people who think like us.

When we overeat, we have plenty of food around, mostly food that we "should not" eat. We cook in large quantities. We eat from large plates and make sure that there is enough food to refill these large plates or bowls.

Sweets Will Do You In

If sweets were given to you as a reward when you were a child, you probably still have sweets stacked away and you will eat them whenever you have the need to reward yourself. The myth of sweets being a reward got you addicted to sugar.

Boredom Will Do You In

Boredom is one of the major reasons for eating. Boredom makes you want to do something. If the only thing you can think of is food, you will eat. You do that usually without paying much attention to what you are doing. Finding something interesting to do will not only make you eat less, it will also be a good remedy for boredom.

Bad Habits Will Do You In

Some people use alcohol or drugs to forget. Some use food to numb their senses. We have that nice sensation of being bad when we eat the food we are not supposed to eat. We are only kidding ourselves. Food can be enjoyed without guilt and can enhance our senses instead of numbing them.

We eat when we go to the movies. It has become a ritual, and the movie industry knows it. A good portion of their income is coming from parading us through the snack food alley on the way to our seat. Despite what you will see on the screen while you are waiting for the movie to start, eating popcorn when you go to the movies is not mandatory.

The list of reasons and opportunities for eating too much food goes on and on.

It is obvious that we have to rearrange a few things before we can embark on a healthy way of eating. We first have to become aware of what is distracting us from following a healthy way of eating and systematically change our surroundings and our social habits. This is important because it is hard to change old habits, and temptations do not make our life easier. We are less tempted to eat if we do not leave food out in the open where we can see it all the time.

Snacks won't bother us if we leave them in the store.

CHAPTER 5

INFORMATION VERSUS MISINFORMATION

What Do Scientists Say?

How do you know if you are listening to a scientist? If you hear somebody say, "You are allowed to eat two from group 1 and only one from group 2," you are probably listening to a nutritional "expert" or you may be getting advice from a waiter in a Chinese restaurant, but it is not likely that you are listening to a nutritional scientist.

Separating information from misinformation in the field of nutrition has become almost impossible. The subject is complex, and the fact that practically anybody can voice an "expert" opinion does not make it any easier. The information explosion, fueled by the Internet, can turn bogus data into widely accepted, factual data because of instant worldwide exposure. The average person, who is looking for legitimate answers to his or her overweight problem, does not have a chance.

Scientific discoveries in recent years indicate that the human body is much more complex than we could ever imagine. Chances are that we have only scratched the surface with our knowledge about the range of nutrients our body utilizes and how the body does it.

If we are not done discovering nutrients, how can we know for sure the effect on our health from the overuse of some foods and particularly the lack of others?

Research findings in the field of nutrition are often supported by studies of the body's response to a single nutritional element. For this research, sometimes less than one hundred people are tested. Half of that group is not tested; they are the control group. The findings will be that a nutrient or food product or a whole group of nutrients or food products are either good or bad for us.

The publication of these findings can, for example, boost or destroy the business of individual companies or whole sections of the food industry. It is probable that the findings of those tests, which do not produce the desired result of the group financing the tests, may never reach the public.

Every human body is basically different from those of others or in a different state of existence. Environmental and emotional conditions have an influence on the state of our body, so does the food we are eating or drinking at any given time.

There are thousands of chemicals approved for human consumptions (drugs, food additives, etc.). There are more and more health food products (vitamins, minerals, herbs, protein powders, power bars, power drinks, etc.) produced, promoted, and sold every day. Health products do not need to be approved for consumption. They are not regulated. Each single organic or chemical item we are ingesting has an effect on the human body. Each combination of any two items that we ingest simultaneously can have a compounded effect. The number of combinations, based on the above, is endless. Therefore, a study of a hundred or even several thousand people can lead to just about any result, depending upon the state of the bodies tested and the results anticipated.

Research is costly. Somebody has to pay for it. Research projects, which can lead to the development of new drugs and new methods of fighting diseases and thereby generate new sources of revenue, are more likely to be funded than nutritional research projects. Research projects that promote health are usually a poor investment for those who are looking for new sources of revenue. Food, occurring in nature, cannot be patented.

The preservation of health therefore becomes the responsibility of each individual.

What Does Everyone Else Say?

Misinformation, misconceptions, and dangerous practices abound in the field of nutrition. The Internet is a playground for off-the-wall opinions and advice. Many people get their nutritional information from the Internet or infomercials financed by those who profit from the sales of the advertised products.

Not a day seems to pass without us being bombarded with advertisements for concoctions that cure us from being relatively healthy (overweight).

When basic needs, such as eating and the desire to control weight, become a playground for the uncontrolled pursuit of profit and human ego, we are in trouble.

Many discoveries in nutritional health have a limited application, limited support data, and are often contradicted by later studies. Nevertheless, modern communication will assure that we learn about these discoveries instantly. Often they cause us to alter our eating habits.

Misinformation becomes mingled with true scientific information and becomes undistinguishable. Although most of us are basically critical, information is handed down from one person to another and soon is considered common knowledge. As a result, we become fearful of the food we like and limit ourselves to foods, which may not provide the nutrients we need and most likely will not bring us any pleasure at all.

At onetime, we knew how and what to eat, and we did not have a weight problem. Then we started to gain weight. Was it because we were told what to eat and what not to eat? At onetime we did not need any food charts to stay healthy. What will happen once we have lost that extra weight? Can we then go back to eating "bad foods?" Bad foods were not an issue before we started to gain weight.

Do not let misinformation scare you from eating. Do not let misinformation cause you to buy products you don't need or that may even be harmful to you. Use your common sense and follow your instincts.

The Danger of Counting Calories

What is a calorie? Is it something to eat? It must be because we are only allowed to eat so many calories a day.

Calories are meaningless to most people. The following demonstrates the danger of artificial dietary rules:

Allow me to become a bit technical. A *calorie* is the metric measurement for the thermal energy needed to increase the temperature of one gram of water by one degree Celsius. Are you following me so far?

Theoretically, we could satisfy our daily allowance of calories by drinking hot water (water with a temperature above that of our body). This interpretation—no matter how logical—is of course ridiculous.

The food and medical industry use the term *calorie* as a measurement for identifying the energy content of food, which can be utilized by the body to keep it warm and flex its muscles.

Calories do not define the nutritional value of any food.

For example, we could and often do eat food that is high in calories, such as cake and anything else that is made from sugar and fat. It does not take a large quantity of this type of food to make us exceed our daily allowance of calories.

Logic tells us that we cannot afford to eat anything else because we have exceeded our daily allowance of calories.

Before we know, cravings kick in. We need something satisfying. We need something "good," and we need it fast because cravings are a type of pain. Forget complex carbohydrates. Forget fruits and vegetables, which take a long time to give us that full feeling and stop the pain. Forget nutritious food. It's back to sugar and fat.

And around and around we go. Therefore, artificial dietary rules can be more dangerous than what they appear to be.

The labeling of foods as "bad" leads us to the exclusion of individual types of food or entire food groups. The recommendation to count calories, as a measure of controlling our food intake, can even be more harmful because it disregards nutritional values.

Nutritious, Unadulterated Food

I state in my hypothesis that eating a large variety of nutritious, unadulterated foods, in small quantities, is the best insurance for getting the proper nutrients and for balancing the body weight. How do we identify nutritious and unadulterated foods?

Any type or category of food comes in different forms. The nutrients available to a plant or an animal during growth will determine their nutrient content. The freshness of the food is also important. Plants, as a rule, reach their highest nutritional potency when they are ripe and lose it when they are starting to spoil.

Food has to be prepared and stored. The preparation and storage of food often depletes it of its nutrients. For example, cooking destroys nutrients that are heat sensitive, and storing or cooking of food in water drains nutrients that are water-soluble.

The nutrient content of processed foods is determined by marketing requirements. These foods have to taste good, look good, and have to be protected against spoilage. Spoilage affects the quality and storability (shelf life) of the food.

This concept does not only apply to prepared foods but also to basic staples like flour. The wheat germ, which is part of a grain kernel, contains a number of nutrients. In some commercially available flour, the wheat germ has been removed. Food products made from this flour, such as pasta, cereals, bread, and other baked goods may therefore contain fewer nutrients than what we would assume.

On the packaging of some processed foods, we find a listing of vitamins and minerals, which may have been added rather than having been preserved as a natural part of the ingredients used. Although vitamins and minerals may be good for us, we may not need those added to the food products; they may have lost their potency during storage and may be of a type that is not easily absorbable by the body.

Table salt is a nutrient the body needs in moderation. Excessive use of salt can be harmful; it can kill you. Many processed foods are loaded with salt because salt enhances the flavor, and it is also a preservative.

It is advisable to educate ourselves about nutrition. Nevertheless, there is more misinformation than serious scientific information floating around.

Learning about nutrients may encourage us to eat a larger variety of foods. The opposite will happen if we let ourselves get scared away from certain foods or whole food groups.

Poisonous food is bad for us. Spoiled food is bad for us. Appearance, aroma, and smell warn us about spoiled food. Spoiled food is usually discolored, has an odor, or tastes bad. If we can't spot spoiled or poisonous food before we eat it, indigestion will let us quickly know. Chemically altered food may be bad for us. Chemical alterations are usually made for the purpose of improving the appearance of processed food and extending its shelf life (masking spoilage). The effect of chemically altered food on our health may not be discovered for years after the food was introduced in the market.

All the other so-called bad foods may only have been maligned. The most common form of maligning food is the attempt of an interest group to gain a market advantage by citing "scientific" evidence that a certain type of food is bad for us. This has led to giving foods a bad name such as fat, eggs, red meat, pork, milk, proteins containing cholesterol (which includes practically all animal products), snacks, fast food, and just about everything else.

Let's be honest. Such foods as chocolate, ice cream, soda, cookies, pastry, candy, and deserts are delightful creations and fun to eat. Cooking with butter makes food taste delicious. Grilled, marbled steaks taste better than those lean cuts. Cream sauces taste delightful. Bacon and sausage are favorites for breakfast.

There is nothing wrong with these foods if eaten in moderation. The only thing wrong is the fact that we are being made to feel guilty for eating them at all. Because we are not supposed to eat them, we are likely to eat them compulsively, whenever our cravings control us.

The occasional use of these foods, in moderate quantities, together with many other foods, may be healthier than what we are made to think. Some of those foods may contain nutrients that have not been discovered yet or their nutritional value has not been properly recognized.

Concentrated nutrients, which can be found in nature such as spices, including salt and acidic foods, can be harmful if not used in moderation. Again, our instincts guide us. Taste and pain protect us from overuse. Caution is warranted. Frequent overuse can numb our senses.

Artificially concentrated nutrients such as distilled alcohol and refined sugar are more treacherous. Taste misleads us. Instead of feeling pain, we feel a sensation of temporary well-being. Refined sugar may well be one of the most innocent looking yet most addictive and harmful concentrated nutrients around. Stay away from sugar if you cannot control it.

Here is a simple but effective formula for selecting foods. Going beyond this basic formula gets complicated.

Eating a large variety of foods in small portions increases the probability that we are supplying the body with a large variety of nutrients, those that are known, as well as those that are still unknown. The more nutrients available to the body in moderation, the more likely it is that the body will stay strong, healthy, painless, and young.

Is Fat Bad for You?

Will those who have been successful in losing and maintaining weight with a low-fat diet alone please stand up!

Among all the information and misinformation about nutrition available, fat seems to be considered the single worst villain that makes us gain weight and is harmful to our health.

The food industry is accommodating us with a large range of low-fat and fat-free foods. These foods usually taste terrible and are priced at a premium. The fact that we now can buy bottled water, advertised as "fat-free," is particularly reassuring.

Fat comes in many forms. Some oils are now considered to be beneficial for the body. Trans fat (also called trans-fatty acids or partially hydrogenated oils) primarily used in margarine (which has long been promoted as a substitute for butter) has now been found to be at least as harmful to your health as butter. Trans fat is also found in breakfast cereals, cupcakes, cookies, candy bars, teething biscuits, and most processed foods that are advertised as low fat. Most low-fat diets are loaded with trans fat.

Doctors prescribe a "low-fat diet" with great authority. But there is no such thing as a single, specific low-fat diet.

The rules for low-fat diets vary widely. Some call for fat being limited to 30 percent of the daily calories consumed. Figuring out how much fat is allowed requires mathematical and food science skills.

One rule limits fat to only 10 percent of the daily food consumption by weight. That appears to be simple. But let me use this rule as a demonstration on how misleading it can be. Assuming a person consumes five pounds of food (including liquids, such as milk and soda) per day. At 10 percent, his fat intake would be a half pound per day. This would be considered a low-fat diet.

This person now starts to follow his instincts and reduces his food intake to one pound (not including liquids like water) per day. He likes fatty foods, and his fat intake occasionally is as high as 25 percent (if that is possible) or one-fourth pound per day.

He would now be considered to be on a high-fat diet in spite of the fact that he effectively cut his fat intake by at least 50 percent a day. He would also not get any credit for choosing the type of oils that are (depending upon the latest research) considered beneficial for the body.

Most low-fat enthusiasts are not aware of the fact that eating fat helps to stay satisfied longer and therefore to eat less.

Low-fat diets have been touted for over thirty years as a sure way to lose weight. They still are in spite of the fact that obesity has steadily increased. Facts don't seem to interfere with nutritional logic.

The Value of Charts and Tables

Any good diet book includes charts and tables about the ideal weight, body shape, calories burned by exercising, and all kinds of data for all kinds of food.

When food charts initially were published, they would tell us how many calories, how much protein, carbohydrates, and fat could be found in basic food items. This information is becoming more detailed and more confusing by the day. The number of food items listed is steadily increasing. They now include prepared and restaurant foods, which frequently change.

We learned that there were different types of fat—bad fat and not so bad fat. Then we learned about cholesterol. We were told that foods containing cholesterol were bad for us (almost all animal products contain cholesterol). Later, we learned that there is more than one type of cholesterol, and some are bad but others are good.

The fact that our body produces its own cholesterol, good and bad, makes it even more confusing to the average person who is eager to escape from this cholesterol trap. And the "average person" is not the only one being confused.

The emergence of enzymes on the nutritional scene further complicated health and weight management efforts. Now it has been discovered that there are still other nutrients that seem to have a strong effect on our health and well-being. Some of these nutrients are called protease inhibitors, oligofructose, pyrroloquinoline quinone, nucleotides, isothiocyanates, conjugated linoleic acid, and so forth. We are bound to find many more nutrients, hopefully with names that are easier to pronounce and to remember.

Eating was made to be a pleasure and not an annoyance. Weight loss diets that require us to analyze every bite we are eating are useless for the average person. Charts and tables with food values are of little help to those who do not purchase and prepare their own food. And that would be the majority of us.

Following our instincts does not require any charts or tables. Ever!

Do You Need Special Recipes?

This book is not just another attempt to sell you overpriced food items. You do not need special recipes, nor do you have to buy any special diet foods. Eat whatever you like, and let your instincts guide you. Use your favorite recipes. Any cookbook will do.

Most recipes offered in diet cookbooks start from the premise that certain foods are bad for you and that you have to maintain a strict eating regimen.

The word *substitute* ranks prominently in diet recipes. Do you really want to eat food substitutes?

Some weight loss diets make it easy for you. You can buy ready-made food. If you don't like that food or you don't buy it, you have a fat chance to succeed (no pun intended).

Some weight loss diets tell you that you can drink your food; you don't even have to chew anymore. Intravenous feeding is presently reserved for medical treatments. But don't despair; it will soon be commercially available as soon as somebody figures out how to get rid of the pole you have to push around to hold the food bag.

What about Vitamins?

I still have a lot of vitamins sitting around. Although most of them are beyond their expiration date, I don't have the heart to throw them out. At onetime or another, they were important to me depending upon whatever book I was reading at that time.

Vitamin supplements make sense as long as we know what they are good for and when we need them. Whenever we cannot eat a large variety of foods or are under stress, vitamins and minerals can be beneficial.

The quality of vitamins varies widely. You may not be getting the vitamins you think you are getting just because they are listed on the packaging. The quantity may be insignificant. They may have lost their potency over time. Your body may not be able to absorb them in the form they are coming. Some vitamins and minerals, particularly herbs, can have a strong effect on your body and serious side effects if you take medication.

Whenever you change your eating habits and enlarge the variety of foods you are eating, there may be some temporary discomfort. Herbs or food supplements can aggravate the situation. If the discomfort continues, you will have to reevaluate what you are doing and consult a doctor.

Be wary of any supplements that claim to reduce weight.

Is Exercise All You Need?

"Exercise (particularly such exercise that makes us spend money) will reduce our weight." Thousands of commercials tell us so every day.

Exercise alone will not reduce our weight unless the energy we get from food is less than the energy we burn.

Exercise is good for your body.

➢ Exercise can be useful; ask anybody who does physical work for a living.
➢ Exercise can be fun; ask anybody who plays sports.
➢ Exercise in a gym can be boring, but it still can be good for you.

Exercise tunes the body and is good for your health. If you use a lot of energy, you have the option to eat more or lose weight. Eating more usually wins.

The body works on the principle "Use it or lose it." This applies to muscles, the brain, and I am sure you can think about some other things. Go for it! Healthy eating habits will give you more energy. An athletic body can carry more weight and will still look good.

It is good to exercise, but exercise alone will not solve your weight problem. Ask a 350-pound linebacker playing football.

Exercise is being touted as a sure way to lose weight. Burning energy has become an obsession for some. There are stimulants available that help us to overextend ourselves physically by inhibiting the bodily indicators of fatigue, all for the sake of losing weight. Those who exercise to lose weight are likely to overdo it. They get weak and hungry and in many cases, eat more.

You do not have to exercise to lose weight. Sensible exercise can help.

The Quality of Life

Medicine is doing a fantastic job in keeping us alive longer. But a longer life is no bargain unless the quality of life does not diminish. Healthy living is the issue, and that is not just important for older people.

The human body has an astonishing capability to repair itself. Physical injuries, smoking, irresponsible use of drugs, alcohol abuse, bad eating habits, and diseases can damage the body; yet in most cases, it still keeps on going or recovers after the abuse stops.

There seems to be no end to the punishment a young body can endure. When we get older, the body becomes less tolerant, and weight gain becomes much easier.

Keeping ourselves healthy is desirable throughout our lives. Once the body is seriously damaged, it may not be able to repair itself completely. Physical damage, drug or alcohol abuse, and diseases can scar the body forever.

Poor nutrition can also damage your body permanently.

Overweight is an indication of poor eating habits. Nevertheless, there is that question, What constitutes overweight?

- As long as overweight does not affect our health, it may not be dangerous.
- As long as overweight does not affect our health and our lifestyle, it may not matter at all.

Being able to control weight is important. Being able to control weight gives us the opportunity to adjust our weight to our needs, medically or otherwise. Temporary weight loss is meaningless and in many cases, unhealthy.

Most weight loss diets have one thing in common; they require a regimen that makes life miserable. Just having to bother with how many calories are in the food we eat, having to buy special foods, having to avoid the foods we like, and having to eat tasteless food is an annoyance and is hard to endure.

Being punished for having gained weight with little hope for pardon is nothing to look forward to.

CHAPTER 6

CONCLUSIONS

Hunger and appetite are natural instincts that keep us well nourished and healthy. Hunger tells us when and how much to eat, and appetite leads us to the foods with the nutritional elements the body needs.

Any interference with our ability to follow those instincts can cause us to become undernourished. The body may simply not get all the nutrients it needs.

Cravings are an indication that the food we are eating does not include all the nutritional elements the body needs. Cravings cause us to keep on eating after our hunger instinct indicates that we are satisfied. It is the body's way to search for the missing nutrients. Cravings interfere with and obstruct the hunger indicator.

If we eat the wrong types of food (foods, which do not include the nutrients the body needs), cravings will most likely make us eat more of the wrong foods. Cravings make us overeat, and overeating is the most common cause of overweight.

Healthy eating habits—following our instincts—will prevent cravings.

Nutritional misinformation, artificial dietary rules, and rigid dietary regimens cause us to limit the range of foods we are eating. Information, which attaches the label *bad* to certain types of foods or whole food groups, will lead us to distrust more and more types of food.

Not being able to eat the foods we like, because we are feeling guilty, will make eating less of a pleasure and impede our appetite (the ability to select the nutrients the body needs). Impeding the appetite instinct will lead to a further reduction of available nutrients. This will, in turn, increase cravings and thereby perpetuate overeating.

Therefore, those weight loss diets, which require an unnatural eating regimen and intentionally or unintentionally cause us to restrict the variety of foods that our appetite tells us to eat, will actually perpetuate obesity.

Simplistic recommendations (such as counting calories) and labeling foods as good or bad mislead us. When we follow weight loss diets that restrict the types of food we are allowed to eat, we replace our natural instincts with unnatural eating regimens. This can lead to serious health problems, especially if we are not under medical supervision.

The way out of this Diet Trap is using common sense and following our instincts. This book makes recommendations on how we can restore healthy eating habits by following our instincts.

CHAPTER 7

ANSWERS TO COMMON QUESTIONS

The following are answers to questions that I have been asked.

➤ **What if I have a diet that works?**

Stay with it. Nevertheless, most weight loss diets work initially but stop working or become unbearable after a while. If you have any doubts, ask yourself these three questions:

1. Do I have fun eating?
2. Is the weight loss diet I am using healthy?
3. Are the eating rules sustainable?

Sincere answers to the first two questions will answer the third one. If eating is not a genuine pleasure (which it should be) or if there is any concern about the effects the diet has on your health, you are setting yourself up for failure. Self-punishment, feeling guilty, or being obese should not become a way of life.

➤ **What about exercise?**

Exercise tunes the body and is good for your health. If you use a lot of energy, you can choose to eat more or to lose weight. The body works on the principle "Use it or lose it." This applies to muscles, the brain, etc. Go for it; healthy eating habits will give you more energy. Why not have more fun while feeling better. An athletic body can carry more weight and will still look good.

Exercise alone will not reduce weight unless the energy you get from the food you eat is less than the energy you spend.

➢ What about vitamins?

Vitamin supplements make sense as long as you know what they are good for and when you need them. Whenever you cannot eat a large variety of food, vitamins and minerals can be beneficial. Some herbs can have a strong effect on your body. Be wary about any supplements that claim to reduce weight.

If you greatly restrict your food intake over a long time, you may not get all the nutrients the body needs. Taking vitamin supplements alone will not be the answer. Use common sense and follow your instincts. Take your time with that weight loss. You will get there as long as you are going in the right direction.

➢ What if I don't succeed?

The only way you can fail is if you never try. Use common sense and let your instincts guide you. Once you experience the pleasure of eating without guilt and once you feel the additional energy you get from healthy eating habits, you may not want to go back to the old habits.

If you did not let your instincts guide you today, so what, there is always tomorrow. Once you got started, chances are you will not overeat anymore because you have learned that you feel better if you eat sensibly. You are now controlling your weight instinctively. Eating sensibly becomes a way of life. You may have heard the expression: "The stomach shrinks."

When you let your instincts guide you, you will learn what works for you and most likely use it in one way or another. As long as you don't make it tough on yourself, like wanting to lose all the weight you gained over years in a couple of weeks, "letting your instincts guide you" is fun.

➢ **What about all those foods that are bad for me?**

Poisonous food is bad for you. Spoiled food is bad for you. Foods that are considered bad for you from time to time may only have been maligned by interest groups. Examples of these are fat, eggs, red meat, carbohydrates, pork, milk, proteins containing cholesterol (which includes practically all animal products), snacks, fast food, and just about everything else.

Any type of food in small portions cannot do much harm. You will know quickly what agrees with you and what does not.

It is definitely more harmful to exclude whole food groups than to eat a large variety of foods in moderation.

➢ **What if I am on medication?**

If you are on medication, let your physician know what you are doing. He needs to know because changing the way you eat may have an effect on the results of his treatment.

If you are overweight, your physician will most likely recommend weight loss. Eating sensibly and a large variety of foods should be healthier than depriving yourself of important nutrients, such as fat, or taking weight loss medication.

➢ **What if I can't be physically active?**

If you are limited in your mobility, an effective and healthy weight management becomes even more important. You do not have to be active to avoid overweight. Your instincts will tell you when, how much, and what to eat. Find ways to keep yourself occupied to avoid the urge to eat because of boredom.

➢ **What if I am pregnant?**

Ideally, the body should be as healthy and fit as possible before becoming pregnant. Once pregnant, it is even more important to be healthy and fit. Pregnancy is not a good time for ambitious weight control. It is also not a good time for limiting the range of nutrients available to the body.

If you know how to control your weight naturally, you may not be overweight when you get pregnant, and you will not have to let worries about gaining too much weight during pregnancy deprive you and your baby's body of important nutrients.

Let your doctor know what you are doing. He will be able to detect deficiencies.

➢ What if I stopped smoking and I have the urge to eat?

Dependencies on cigarettes or other drugs often go along with being nutritionally undernourished. Cravings during withdrawal seem to indicate that. Expanding the variety of foods you eat and taking time to enjoy eating are the best ways to stop the cravings. If you know how to lose weight naturally, a temporary weight gain is not a catastrophe. Medical advice is recommendable.

➢ What if I love chocolate, ice cream, and other "bad" foods?

There is nothing bad about chocolate, ice cream, soda, and those other bad foods. The only thing bad is the way some of us overuse them.

I personally love chocolate and ice cream and those other bad foods. I eat them once in a while, but I make a conscious effort to limit the amount. I usually don't keep these foods in the house, and I make sure that eating these foods does not become a compulsion.

➢ What if I lose too much weight?

You may be following your instincts without having fun. Paying attention when you eat, chewing well, decorating your plate, and eating a great variety of food that you like, or get to like, makes eating fun again and weight control easy. If you want to lose weight, stop eating when the hunger stops. If you want to balance your weight, you may eat more liberally.

> ### What if I am too busy?

There are periods when we are involved in activities or work that cause us to be anxious, nervous, or tense.

Don't panic. As long as this way of life does not become a bad habit, it will pass. In the meantime, do as well as you can under the circumstances.

Intestinal pains will remind you that you are doing something wrong. If you have learned to know better, you will notice those pains and respond.

> ### What if food is the only thing that makes me feel good?

You are in luck. Chewing your food well and eating a large variety of food in moderation will make you feel better than ever before. The sensation of not having the "pain of being full" and not feeling guilty may alone make a difference.

Don't get satisfying your cravings mixed up with the pleasure of eating. Cravings hurt. Eating to satisfy cravings is trying to stop a pain. Eating can be a real pleasure if you follow your instincts.

> ### What if it is too hard to get started?

It is not a matter of *starting*; it is a matter of *stopping* bad eating practices. Eating a large variety of foods, in small portions, whenever you are hungry is not something that takes a lot of willpower. You can ease into it.

You will have to get rid of distractions and bad habits. The only way you can be unsuccessful is by not trying.

Enjoying your food, never being hungry, and not being in pain from overeating will make you feel good and will give you more energy. Once you have experienced this feeling, you will want it to last.

Those who are searching for answers in a world abundant with misleading information may find them by joining the non-profit organization The Common Sense Cause. It provides a forum for those who are motivated by humanitarian concerns and believe in the moral responsibility of assisting the general public in pursuing practical and common sense solutions in the field of nutrition and the preservation of health.

Write to:

The Common Sense Cause
P.O Box 2220
Cherry Hill, NJ 08034-0167
commonsensecause@aol.com